MW01688564

Down (Syndrome) But Not Out

A Journey from Grief to Joy

Joyce Sampson

Pleasant Word
A Division of WINEPRESS PUBLISHING

Pleasant Word (a division of WinePress Publishing, PO Box 428, Enumclaw, WA 98022) functions only as book publisher. As such, the ultimate design, content, editorial accuracy, and views expressed or implied in this work are those of the author.

ISBN 13: 978-1-4141-0806-3
ISBN 10: 1-4141-0806-0
Library of Congress Catalog Card Number: 2006907198

Dedication

It is with great joy that I, along with my husband, Bill, dedicate this book to our younger son, Kerry. We are so blessed and grateful that God chose to place you in our home. Your integrity and humor are a constant delight to us. Thank you for being the fine person you are!

Table of Contents

Acknowledgements

I'd like to say thanks to:

My husband, Bill, who has been my source of encouragement through the writing of this manuscript. He is my best friend, my confidante, my life's partner of forty-six years and my joy of life.

My sis, Janice, who critiqued this manuscript in its early stages. Thanks for your input and for coming to our aid several times in the past to care for Craig in our absence. You enabled Bill and me to slip away for a wonderful cruise, leaving Craig in your capable hands for a week. What a memory!

Our former neighbors, Peggy and Jerry, who instantly loved Craig, unconditionally, and made their home a safe harbor for those times when Craig needed another set of parents.

My long-time friends, Carol, Joyce and Joyce (Mum-mum) who provided me with love, support, a listening ear, and a few days' rest and relaxation in Florida each year for the past sixteen years.

Our next-door neighbor, Judy, who gave her professional advice, direction, and encouragement.

Craig's grandparents, Darl, Evelyn, and Edna, and his pseudo grandparents, Stanley and Trudy, who gave so generously of their time and so sincerely of their prayers.

Ada Johnson, our dear friend, who shared her expert writing advice, critique, encouragement and above all, her prayers.

Dr. Travis Collins, our Pastor, who read the manuscript, prayed and encouraged us in this project.

Prologue

Craig William Sampson, weighing a mere five and a half pounds, made his entrance into the world three weeks ahead of schedule on September 23, 1966, in Lima, Ohio. A few days later, I, his mother and the narrator of this story, and my husband, Bill, were given a tentative diagnosis of his condition, called Mongolism at that time (a term which has, mercifully, been replaced by Down syndrome). Down syndrome is a congenital disorder caused by the presence of an extra chromosome in which the affected person has mild to moderate mental retardation. In Craig's case his condition was diagnosed as translocation, a chromosomal problem in which an extra chromosome is attached to another chromosome in each of the cells in his body. This occurs in only 2-3% of children born with Down syndrome.

I immediately began to search for literature and support groups that would both enlighten and encourage us regarding this disorder. Dale Evans Roger's delightful little book, *Angel Unaware,* was the only reading source available other than technical books. Parental support groups, unfortunately, were all too often a pooling of negative emotions regarding their children.

As time went on I began to sense a need to share the story of Craig's journey in this life with others with the thought that some parent, relative or friend of a special needs person may either relate to or be encouraged by our experiences. My purpose in writing these memoirs is not only to uplift others, but also to illustrate the sustenance and support that we have received from our families, our friends, our neighbors, and especially from God. Our faith is the guiding force and strength of our lives, and it is inseparable from who we are. We make no apology for that; we want to share the love we have enjoyed. The sadness that enveloped our lives on September 23, 1966, has disappeared. You will feel the transformation as you read along. In place of sadness we have come to realize that God gave us a special gift. Craig brings love and humor to our home on a daily basis. We are forever changed because of him.

Chapter 1

The Arrival

The morning was overcast and gloomy, and as the two doctors approached my hospital bedside, I sensed a foreboding. When the general practitioner and the pediatrician gently broke the news that our three-day-old baby, for whom we had waited seven years, displayed many signs of Down syndrome, my mind seemed to freeze, unwilling to accept what was said, or to give up our hopes and dreams of a healthy child. A panorama of those dreams flashed through my mind–our son growing, speaking, achieving, attending college, and getting married. Somehow I had to accept the fact that these milestones might never be reached.

Yet our loving God, who promised never to forsake us, had carefully prepared my husband, Bill, and me for the special son He was placing in our home. Both of us had been raised in Christian homes and as children had come to believe in Christ. My personal goals in life had always been clear-cut: first, to seek the partner who was *the one* for me; second, to establish a home based upon Godly precepts and service; and third, to train our children "in the way they should go" (1). Our faith was, still is, and always will be an integral part of our lives. God allowed many tests and Master-instructed us before He was satisfied that this home was prepared for one of His more precious gifts.

In the spring prior to graduation from high school, Bill and I began dating. After graduating and starting our careers, we became aware the two of us shared similar priorities and purposes in life. On a cold, crisp Valentine's Day in 1960, we were married in the presence of many friends and family in a church wedding in Ohio.

Nearly seven years passed before the Lord began to fulfill the third aspect of my goals. After dealing with infertility issues, correcting minor medical problems and experiencing the disappointment of several miscarriages, the news came once again that we were to become parents. Elated beyond measure Bill and I began preparing for the child that was to bless our home. Then at the first trimester of my pregnancy, fear struck as I was rushed to the hospital in an effort to avoid another dreaded miscarriage. I shall never forget the comfort and gentle understanding of our doctor as he bent over me and explained that the chances of carrying this baby full-term were now only twenty-five percent. Even in the turmoil of those moments, however, God's promise that with Him "all things are possible" (2) filtered through the confusion of my emotions and filled me with His peace.

Wondrously, the crisis passed and I was discharged from the hospital. The succeeding weeks were a beautiful interlude of peaceful rest in anticipation of the birth of our child. How nice it would be if all mothers-to-be could experience such an interval before the arrival of their children–a time to prepare for the truly awesome tasks ahead.

On a beautiful fall morning in September we made the momentous trip to the hospital. By evening we were parents of Craig, a sweet 5-1/2 pound boy, born three weeks prematurely. Family and friends who had been praying faithfully for several months shared these happy first days with us. It seemed like a culmination—an end-of-the-journey experience. Little did we realize that it was only the beginning of an uncharted trip! Being a brand new mother, how was I to know that my tiny baby's constant, deep sleeping, his inability to take nourishment, his limpness, and general lethargy were warning signs to the doctors and nurses?

Chapter 2

In My Distress I Cried....

Slowly, the doctors' words began to penetrate my mind and Bill and I began a progression through the various steps of grief. DENIAL: "No, the diagnosis of Down syndrome cannot be true! The outward signs of Down syndrome can be explained away as various family traits." ANGER: "We waited seven years for our first-born. Why must this happen?" BARGAINING: "The extra care and protection of a handicapped child will hinder us from serving you, Lord." DEPRESSION: When Bill and I came to this stage, only God, in all His love and grace, could draw us together and lift us out of our deep despair. This was the mountain we had to climb. At times depression and discouragement threatened to overwhelm me. In 1967 there was a definite lack of literature, support groups, and programs at the disposal of Down's families. I craved support and understanding as I held my tiny baby, rocking and crying.

The Bible became my source of comfort and support, and the fourth chapter of Philippians in particular took on new meaning as God's promises to supply our needs and our strengths became a vital reality. Family, friends, neighbors, and church families poured out love and encouragement, yet I still fought the enemy of depression.

One wintry evening I was feeling especially alone. Bill was attending a church meeting, and Craig was snuggled in his crib for the night. Snow fell outside and the house was cozy and quiet, but a battle raged within me. It was time to get this matter resolved within myself and defeat the enemy that sapped my energy. My piano, untouched for many weeks, seemed to beckon me. As I sat down and ran my fingers over its dusty keys, a desire to hear some of the old beloved hymns arose. Turning the pages of the hymnal, I began to play and sing, "All to Jesus, I surrender (1). I shuffled the pages and stopped and sought a new song, "Have Thine Own Way, Lord" (2). A lump arose in my throat and tears filled my eyes as I began song after song, unable to sing the words of commitment without a deep wrenching from within. As the tears flowed unchecked, I bowed my head at the keyboard, sobbing and praying, asking Christ to remove all traces of self-desire from my life and conform my will to His in total acceptance and submission.

How much time God and I spent together that evening in close communion, I have no concept. However, I vividly recall rising from the piano bench with a peace in my heart and a new song. God uses many means to stimulate our growth–His Word, prayer, circumstances, etc.–but the ministry of Christian music has been particularly meaningful to me since that evening. It is my constant prayer that He will use me as He chooses in this area.

Although our fervent prayer had been that the doctor's tentative diagnosis would prove wrong, it was not to be. When our son, Craig, was 4-1/2 months old, the doctor confirmed his original diagnosis and we were ready for:

ACCEPTANCE! (3) "Giving thanks always for ALL things unto God and the Father in the name of our Lord Jesus Christ" (4) …AND HE HEARD ME!" (5).

Chapter 3

Beginning The Journey

"Jesus wants Craig for a sunbeam, to shine for him each day...." (1). Music became the tool used to cajole our baby into eating, to quiet him for a nap, and to calm his fears. Mothers of Down's children quickly realize how much their little ones love and respond to music. Oh, how I sang as I spooned (and re-spooned) baby food into his resolute little mouth, and coaxed milk down his tiny throat. Due to his flaccid musculature, feedings were laborious, time-consuming tasks. Craig usually required an hour to consume 2-1/2 ounces of formula. The 2:00 a.m. feedings were particularly challenging, and my head bent over his more often than not as we slept through bottle time together. Bill helped out with the nightly routine on weekends, which was a tremendous help to me.

Winter brought its usual viruses and flu epidemics, and we soon learned that Down syndrome babies are especially susceptible to upper respiratory infections. Craig began catching colds in September and was seldom free of them until April, at which time he would go into an early spring allergy, lasting until mid-July. In January of Craig's first year, I came down with influenza. A few days later Craig became ill. His temperature soared to 106 degrees and we feared convulsions or brain damage. I am convinced the Lord occasionally allows sickness in our lives to serve His purposes. It was certainly a time of testing and assessment for us. We realized the depth of love we already felt for our child. Many anxious hours were spent rocking, praying and, yes, singing. When Craig's fever finally broke, we wept unabashedly.

When our doctor confirmed his original diagnosis of Down syndrome, we renewed our dedication of Craig to the Lord. The ups and downs of the coming months tore at our vitality and strength, but they never shook our love for him. We knew from that moment on we would advocate for his medical care, his educational training and his acceptance in the community. Little did we know that all three concerns would be greatly challenged.

Chapter 4

From the Baby Book

"To everything there is a season, and a time to every purpose under the heavens."

—Eccl. 3:1 (1)

Craig's baby book reveals a time schedule of its very own. Differing sharply from the norm, it was God's timing for the development of this special little boy.

Pulls self up and stands alone–24 months. Crawls–17 months. Takes first step alone–3 years, 9 months. First tooth–13 months. Several lines remain blank to this day, such as Gallops and Skips and Laces shoes. Yet from the pages of the baby book emerges a unique personality of an outgoing, lovely, loving and loved baby.

Craig moved through the stages of babyhood slowly, taking time to savor every moment of his infancy, thus making it many months longer than the usual. At times he seemed to remain on a plateau of development indefinitely; then he would slowly inch forward again. Normal children progress much the same way, leveling off at times. The difference is that the developmentally delayed child's progression is in slow motion; the leveling-off intervals are more apparent.

By the time Craig was eighteen months old, we had become weary of the rounds of colds, influenza, and bronchitis, and discouraged with the effort of taking Craig with us everywhere. Each exposure to the public during cold and flu season meant running risks of further illnesses. But those risks had to be weighed against the lack of stimulation that would result from isolating him from others.

Fortunately a county home trainer, Mrs. Goist, was introduced to us. She scheduled weekly visits in our home, the first step of Craig's formal educational experience. These one-hour sessions proved to be invaluable as she introduced him to developmental toys and assisted me in grappling with various problems. Her first advice was, "Don't stop taking Craig with you shopping, going to church, visiting friends, attending ballgames. Each exposure to these activities provides much-needed stimulation for the handicapped child." So we continued our active schedule, including Craig, but I must admit that I was tempted to grab him and head for the nearest exit every time someone sneezed!

As people touched his life and broadened his horizons, so he touched and enlarged their capacity to give and reach out to the handicapped. When Craig escaped the confines of our house with regularity, he grew to love people and in turn usually received love and acceptance from them. In a few short months, he was transformed into an outgoing, friendly little boy, and learned to adjust to changes in his routine–to *flex* as we called it. I cannot begin to name all the friends and neighbors who reached out to us with encouragement during this time. Sales associates in malls would stop and talk to Craig, watching him while I shopped. Caring friends at church took care of him when we arrived, enabling me to worship without interruption, to teach in Sunday school, and participate in the music ministry. Teenagers were especially attentive to him, and he really thrived on their attention. Offers from them to babysit literally poured in. And my mother made a point of grandma-sitting with Craig one morning a week, freeing me to shop, go to the beauty salon, and other necessary things. God was answering our prayers and providing His strength and comfort through His people. There truly was "... a time to weep and a time to laugh" (2).

Unhappy moments? Yes, there were many. The prolonged stares of inquisitive children were often difficult to handle. Craig was too small to notice their excessive curiosity, but I was often distressed. However, as public awareness of developmentally challenged people increased, young mothers began stepping up to use those moments to instruct their children about special needs people. In addition I learned to quickly assess the situation and introduce Craig to other children if the setting seemed appropriate. Occasionally the only way to successfully get past the moment was to pick Craig up and remove him from the scene.

Being a naturally impatient person, I was often discouraged by the slowness of Craig's development, particularly in large motor areas such as crawling, climbing, and walking. Unfortunately when one asks God for patience it does not arrive in a gift-wrapped box. As I pleaded with the Lord for more patience, He answered by teaching me daily to be calm and trust Him even in the most trying situations. At times I wanted to stomp my foot and cry, "*Now*, Lord! I need patience *Now*!" However, Christ's beautiful examples of *His* patience with *me* were the lessons I needed.

In spite of the physical impairments of a Downs child, Craig had little difficulty learning to talk. Following the advice of a speech therapist, I prepared picture scrapbooks, with one picture per page, for Craig. As he mastered a new word, I would add that word, pictorially, as a page to the book. Thus he retained his vocabulary in each review of the growing scrapbook. I was advised never to correct his pronunciation, but to smile, look him in the eye and say the word back slowly and correctly. He

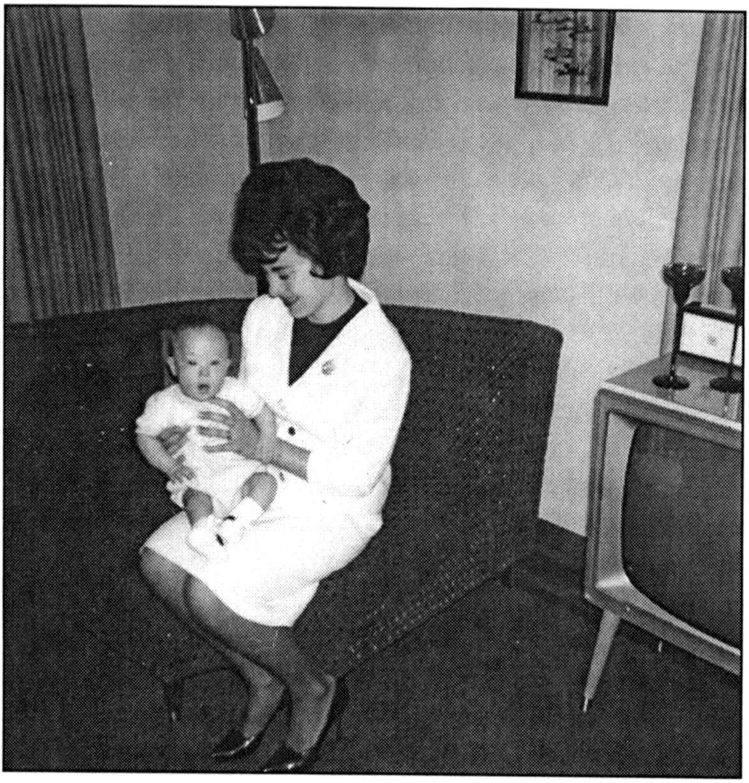

Joyce holding eight-month-old Craig

was always delighted that we had recognized his version and soon corrected himself. Some of his most stirring words will be shared with you.

Chapter 5

From Early Intervention to Early School

Slowly the white station wagon, bearing the name *Marimor School*, turned the corner and started up our driveway. Holding Craig in my arms, I approached the car with a certain degree of reluctance—all right, a *lot* of reluctance! The driver flashed me an understanding smile as she reached for Craig, and promised to personally look after him to and from school–a promise she kept for many years. (Thank you, Lord, for people like the Pohlabels who devoted their time, energy and love to provide for and protect our children).

The days of the home trainer were behind us now. Early Intervention, a program facilitated by the county in which we lived, was designed to expose pre-school developmentally challenged children to classes for abbreviated periods, two or three days a week. At this point Craig was not yet three-years-old and was non-ambulatory, but he thrived on the stimulation school afforded and adjusted readily to his new surroundings and schedule. I did not do as well. The value of early intervention, however, has been documented repeatedly, and these programs have improved tremendously over the years.

From Early Intervention, Craig then progressed to daily attendance at Marimor School, a school for special needs persons, where he remained for several years until his dad's job transferred the family to another city. Craig's daily education was formed under the auspices of an I.E.P. (Individualized Educational Plan), which was drawn up and reviewed annually. This important document was the blueprint for all the services he would receive–occupational therapy, speech therapy, etc. Each year, we realized more and more how crucial the I.E.P. was. Craig's goals and aims needed to be carefully thought out and expressed in this document, for it was a legal instrument and the guideline to which his teacher would refer on a daily basis. As parents, we learned to become watchdogs of that important document. Needless to say the quality of his education rested squarely upon the shoulders of his teachers. Before leaving that city we, along with his dynamic teacher, crusaded for a comprehensive reading program to be established in the school. There were many students who were capable of learning to read more than the survival words being currently taught. After meeting with the 169 Board of Education and presenting our opinions, we finally received approval. The new reading program was purchased and installed, but bogged down when the supporting teacher left two years later.

Interestingly the memory that Craig cherishes regarding his years at Marimor School has virtually nothing to do with the special education process. Rather it encompasses a small trophy that resides in Craig's box of treasures which reads, "Best Halloween Costume, Marimor School, 1974". Honestly, there were years in which I went all out to create a Halloween costume, whipping up astronaut, cowboy and football costumes on my trusty Singer sewing machine. That particular year, however, was not one of those times. In a last-ditch effort to produce a costume for Craig, I dressed him in my wig, a skirt, a red shawl, and gave him a basket to carry. He was quite a picture with his bright brown eyes, black hair and rosy cheeks. Then I sent Little Miss Red Riding Hood off to school.

When Craig returned home that afternoon, bearing the trophy and a big smile, I was amused. However, before I'd had an opportunity to explain all this to Bill, he, in the home of a client, saw Craig in full costume on the televised 6:00 p.m. news. His first-born son in a wig and a skirt. And he was less than amused!

Chapter 6

The Tow-Headed Blue-Eyed Miracle

In the middle of Craig's third year a miracle occurred. It arrived wrapped in a little blue blanket and contained a noisemaker, which often disturbed the peace of the household and forced Craig to share his space on the Sampson pedestal. The arrival of this little towhead capped off six months of prayerful anticipation.

As a result of genetic testing regarding translocation (1), my husband and I had been informed that Craig's condition was hereditary and the likelihood of our having another child with Down syndrome was rather high–between twenty-five and thirty-three percent. While we dearly loved our Down's child, we did not think it wise to take this risk. Adoption was the avenue we chose to increase our family. And God had a child waiting for our home.

Kerry, Craig's new brother, joined the loving arms of our household in June, 1969, and Craig's life was never the same thereafter; it was changed for the better! We watched Craig's reaction to his new baby brother go from rejection, to tolerance, to delight. Here was a live-in partner with whom he could crawl about, giggle and explore. By the time Kerry had reached eight months, I was referring to the boys as our wrecking crew. Kerry taught Craig all sorts of new tricks—how to climb stairs, open doors and drawers and upend wastebaskets, even how to walk.

I had literally worn out my jeans, crawling backwards around the floor encouraging Craig to walk on his own. I knew he could accomplish this feat, even though he was double-jointed and quite unsteady on his feet. But it wasn't until Kerry took his first steps and basked in the applause and hugs of his grandparents that Craig announced, "I can walk, too!" And he did. Right across the room and into his grandmother's arms. What an unforgettable evening. A double blessing!

As little boys, Craig and Kerry loved to *be* together even though they were too young to *play* together. Often, they stood back-to-back in parallel play, seemingly ignoring one another, but anxious to find the other if he disappeared for even a moment.

For several years I was concerned how their relationship would be affected when Kerry surpassed Craig in size, functional ability and sociability. Looking back, I scarcely recall how and when it happened. Their roles in life simply changed, each accepting and supporting the other, and the transition went quite smoothly. Craig's greatest fan as he participated in Special Olympics was his brother who coached, cheered, and attended every event. Likewise as Kerry played sports all through his school years, Craig was his loyal fan, rarely taking his eyes off his brother.

When Kerry began driving a car, Craig was not easily convinced that his buddy could handle this new accomplishment. Shortly after Kerry received his driver's license, I sent the two out to pick up a pizza. The plan was for Kerry to drive and Craig to hold the pizza. When they returned Kerry came in carrying the pizza while Craig slowly climbed out of the car. It seemed that Craig, white-knuckled, could not let go of the armrest and the door handle long enough to hold the pizza!

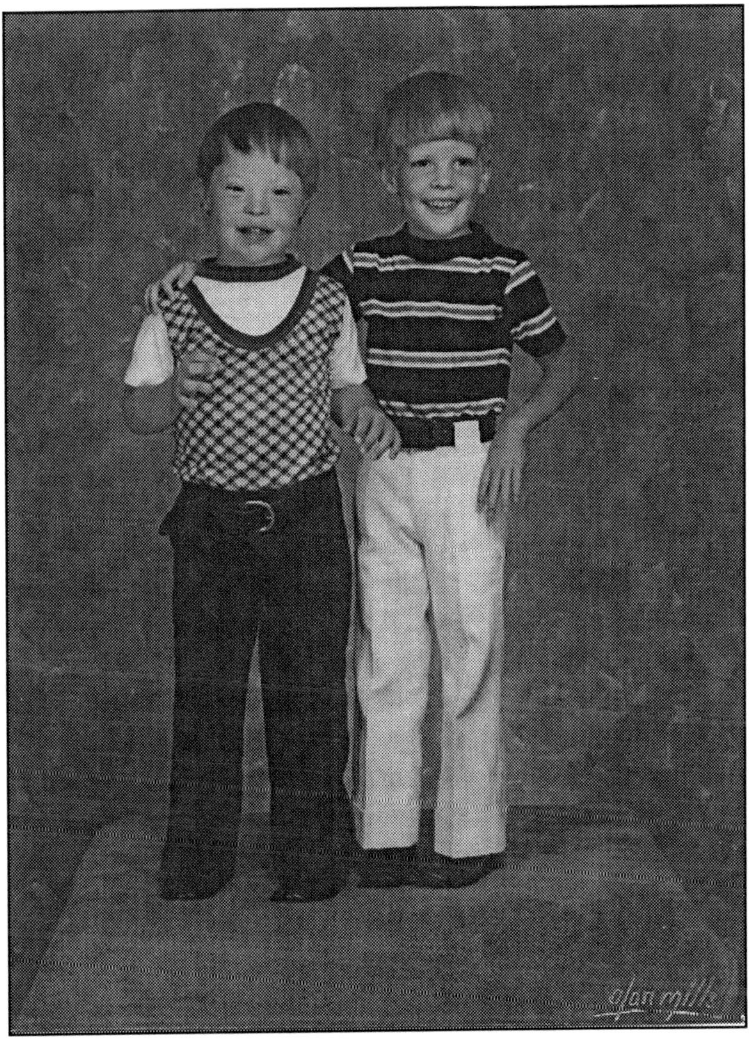

Craig and Kerry – Best Pals

Kerry's early school writings reflected a growing protectiveness for his brother. I also noticed that as he grew up, his friends had to relate well to Craig–or they did not remain friends for very long. Now in adulthood Kerry remains very tuned in to his brother. He understands Craig's speech, senses his frustrations, and makes himself available to support and assist his brother.

The year before Kerry married, he spent several months living at home, assisting with Bill's recovery from open-heart surgery. Early one morning, as Craig stood beside the driveway waiting for the van to pick him up and transport him to work, he became light-headed and fell to the ground, fainting and cutting his face on the concrete. Kerry scooped him up (while a protesting Craig awoke and insisted that he was going to work), cleaned his face and bundled him into the car for a trip to the nearest hospital. After spending twelve hours waiting with his parents in the emergency room, Craig was finally admitted to the hospital's cardiac ward for further tests. Mother and Dad were exhausted by this time and decided to go home and rest. But Kerry was unwilling to leave Craig alone and he spent the night in a chair beside his bed. The next morning Craig was dismissed from the hospital, none the worse except for a few stitches on his face.

Throughout the years I have noticed that siblings of special persons often develop maturity beyond their years, along with an intensified sensitivity and understanding for those who may have vulnerabilities. Clearly Kerry is a different person because of Craig. Conversely Craig is a different person because of Kerry. Their influence upon one another has been remarkable.

At the time of this writing, Craig is joyously welcoming another member into our family—his sister-in-law, Amy. She tells me that Kerry filled her in on Craig as they walked the beach on one of their first afternoons together. From the time Amy threw the bouquet at their wedding to her new brother-in-law, through her studying him and his special likes (primarily Pringles), she has become a wonderfully positive force in his life. Her growing understanding of special needs persons as she encounters them in the classroom and school where she teaches is a positive force in their lives as well. I know the parents of these special needs students have grown to respect and love Amy–but not nearly as much as we do!

I have moved ahead several years in my narration; let's return to Craig's early years and resume our story.

Chapter 7

A Bit of Love, A Handshake, A Hug

Chubby, soft, expressive hands—designed and used for giving to others—were tenderly resting on my forehead as I battled a raging migraine one stifling summer afternoon. Craig's solicitude was slightly overwhelming, and when he disappeared from the room, I must admit that I felt greatly relieved. Unable to leave the boys unsupervised to retreat to the quiet of my room, I had sprawled on the family room floor, trying to subdue the throbbing in my head. Moments later Craig reappeared with his pillow in hand and brought it to me, placing my head on it and soothing me with his funny little pats. He then rejoined his brother to watch television, and I smiled to myself thinking what a dear, sweet child he is.

Ten minutes later Craig was peering over me, waking me and asking if my headache was better now. I smiled my sweetest at him and assured him, somewhat untruthfully, that it was much better. He replied, "Good!" and removed the pillow with one decisive movement, leaving me blinking and dumbfounded, whereupon he retreated to the television once more, enthroned now upon his pillow. In spite of the strange things going on inside my head, I was forced to chuckle.

The hands of a Down's child are usually open in an attitude of giving, consoling, and aiding others. How many times did I see him bend over my dear mother as she courageously struggled through the throes of cancer and gently pat her shoulder, assuring her of his love and need of her? And how sweet to hear her confide that Craig was often her inspiration to keep on battling that long summer years ago.

How many times his hand brushed away a tear, reached for a hug, offered a handshake to a bereaved one? A sixth sense, you may say, a compensation—or do these persons possess a capacity for love beyond our human understanding? Perhaps they see a world few people get to see.

At this writing, Craig is thirty-nine years old. He still slips up behind my chair and places his hand on my forehead when I have admitted to no one that I have a headache. His tenderness towards people and his awareness of their needs remind me of the words of Luke, the beloved physician of the New Testament: "these hands have ministered unto my necessities and to them that were with me" (1).

Chapter 8

So Who Needs Hair?

When Craig was around five years of age, his hair began to fall out in small, quarter-sized spots at first, gaining momentum rapidly until the loss was complete. During this time I questioned our pediatrician about Craig's lethargy, his dry skin, his loss of hair, his hoarse voice. Thyroid imbalance was an obvious conclusion to me, but the doctor didn't seem to take my opinions seriously. Much later Craig was diagnosed with hypothyroidism (and I learned how to assertively advocate!). Correction of this thyroid problem resulted in dramatic improvements in skin tone, hoarseness of voice, stamina and height; in fact, he grew twelve inches in height over the next three years. However, Craig's hair never returned and we had to resort to the use of full hairpieces.

Understating this whole experience, Craig was not fond of wearing these hairpieces, although he complied for church, school, and social outings. Immediately upon returning home he would remove his hairpiece, peeling it back as though he were being scalped, and toss it on the stairs. At home he usually wore a favorite blue fishing hat–or not. Concerned about shocking others, especially children, I kept a close watch on this behavior until the doorbell rang one day just moments after Craig had returned home from school. The paperboy had come to collect, I was in another part of the house, and I heard Craig open the front door. Realizing that his hair probably now lay in plain view on the steps, I rounded the corner and started down the steps at full speed. Just then I heard the paperboy ask, "What happened to your hair?" Craig drew himself up to his full fifty-eight inches of height, placed his hands on his hips, and replied, "So who needs hair?"

Later in life, Craig was to deal with severe allergies and acid reflux issues, but I never again doubted his ability to stand up for himself. God had planted a healthy measure of resiliency in him.

The blue fishing hat, which we now refer to as ole' blue, is a story in itself. The cherished hat still exists today, having been repeatedly laundered, mended, sold and bought back again. Nothing can replace it—neither denim, khaki nor corduroy. It now conforms perfectly to the contours of its owner's head and is soft as a glove, but it is the history, its past, that makes ole' blue irreplaceable.

Many years ago a friendship was forged that blossomed with this little blue hat. One summer morning I was holding Craig in my arms as we slowly exited the church sanctuary following the morning service. Directly in front of me stood this man, his attractive wife and three lovely daughters, visitors to our small church for the first time. Brice stood some six feet, five inches tall and his size must have intimidated me, because I remember telling myself that I *should* greet this man and welcome him and his family. At that very moment, however, Craig simply reached around Brice, grabbed his arm and said hello. It was the beginning of a beautiful friendship that lasted until Brice's sudden death in 1996.

Brice loved that little blue hat and helped himself to it on occasion, but could only enjoy wearing it momentarily because

Craig literally crawled up Brice to retrieve it. One day he offered to buy the hat and flashed fifty cents in front of Craig. Craig, ever the astute businessman, readily accepted the offer and the deal was consummated. For about five minutes. Realizing his folly, Craig then began the retrieval process.

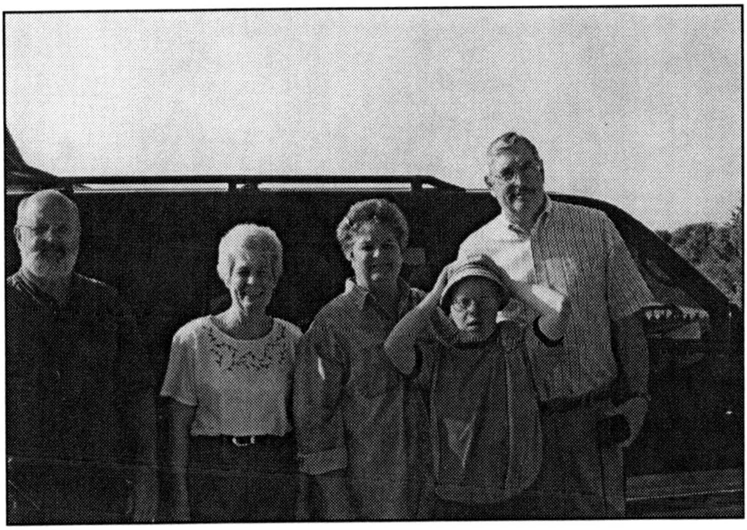

Ron, Joyce, Carol, Brice and Craig, protecting ole' blue

This game repeated itself for years; the stakes even rose to one dollar. In all the episodes, Craig always wound up both richer and in possession of ole' blue.

It is the story of turning a calamity into a victory.

Chapter 9

It's Rude To Snore!

Living in a quiet cul-de-sac among friendly neighbors, Craig was able to move comfortably up and down Kingsbury Court at our Lima home, seeking companionship with neighbors when he got bored with things around home. As parents we were paying close attention to the development of his social skills in an effort to help him develop his own circle of friends. Occasionally, however, our well-meaning efforts just downright flopped.

One summer afternoon I realized that Craig had been gone from our house longer than was comfortable for me. Just as I started out the door to search for him, the phone rang. It was our neighbor two doors down the street, the home of three teenage daughters who regularly showered Craig with attention. They wanted to let me know where he was and that they'd like him to stay and visit for a while.

A little later Craig returned home, looking very pleased with himself. Then the phone rang again. It seems that the girls' father, Mr. Darbyshire, had returned home from work and stretched out, still in his suit and tie, on the easy chair to take a nap—a daily ritual. But his ritual was different this time because Craig was there. After he had fallen into a deep sleep and had begun to snore lightly, Craig woke him up and informed him that it was rude to snore! I made sure that Craig did not go calling at that hour again.

The poet, John Donne, had it right when he wrote, "No man is an island." The neighbors who have surrounded our homes in the various cities in which we have lived have been most kind and supportive and have not left us stranded. The first city in which we lived, Lima, Ohio, had been a railroad town at the turn of the twentieth century, the home of Lima Locomotive Works. Thus, its streets were crossed with railroad tracks–tracks that bore trains, which made one late for appointments and late getting back home before the school bus arrived. It was great to have neighbors who watched out for each other's children and readily opened their doors as a haven of safety–even at the risk of having their naps interrupted.

Chapter 10

You Know I Hate Meatloaf–and Other Prayers

One of the highlights of Christian parenting is the privilege of listening in on your child's prayers. We've gained insights into the thinking of our boys and discovered many truths about them as we bowed our heads before meals. Sore throats that would not be admitted to Mother (lest she ban swimming for that day), grouchy dispositions (again, directed at Mother), and sweet concerns for grandparents, Sunday school teachers, and neighbors were revealed in those precious moments. Craig seems to have his own special line to God, and uses it whenever and wherever he feels the need. Many poignant moments have been created as he called the Lord's attention to someone's needs. But there was one occasion when he felt compelled to complain a little to God.

My meatloaf recipe tends to conform to whatever leftovers need to be cleared out of the refrigerator; consequently, meatloaf for dinner at our house indicates that it is grocery shopping time. This is not Craig's favorite entrée by far, and my announcement that meatloaf is on the menu usually brings several groans from him, along with much pressure to "*Please*, let's have hotdogs, pizza or spaghetti!" One evening as we bowed heads to ask the

Lord's blessing upon our meatloaf dinner, Craig fervently prayed, "Lord, *please* bless Mommy and help her get to the grocery store tonight. You know I *hate* meatloaf!" Needless to say, it was several months before I could bring myself to serve meatloaf again.

For many years as our sons grew up, Bill and I functioned as volunteer teen directors at our church. What a wonderful world of opportunities this opened up for Craig and Kerry. They attended the weekly Bible studies and most of the parties, which usually included pizza, Craig's all-time favorite food. If we needed babysitters there was a waiting list–Michele, Laura, Barb, and Becky to name a few. They were great with both of the boys, and opened up their world to lots of teenage fun–football games, music contests, swimming, and even high school musicals.

Our local high school rehearsed and presented musicals in the spring of each year, which I sometimes accompanied on the piano. This necessitated taking the boys to many rehearsals, offering them opportunities to get acquainted with even more teenagers. These young people enjoyed interacting with our boys and often treated them to goodies from the corner mom and pop store. As a result of these rehearsals, Craig became very familiar with the songs and lines in "Fiddler on the Roof" (1), memorizing both the script and the music. He especially loved Golde's famous line, "Do I *What*?" which he tried out on me occasionally. In fact, Craig had memorized both the speaking lines and the songs so well that Bill, noticing his lips moving all through the opening performance, frequently had to remind him not to speak or sing aloud.

Our doors were always open to young people, and they stopped frequently on their way to and from work and school. Two of Craig's cousins, Julie and Debbie, were able to participate in the teen group during their summer vacations. Their impact upon Craig was immense and he thoroughly enjoyed the attention they gave him. He knew all the other teens by name, where they attended school, who was dating whom, and what their favorite football team was (not necessarily in that order).

One evening as we closed a family devotional with prayer, we prayed specifically, as always, for each teen, mentioning them by name and lifting up their unique needs and requests. Just as Bill said "Amen," Craig added his P.S: "God, don't forget Mimi!" It seemed that we had inadvertently omitted one of thirty some young people—a lovely girl named Mimi. To this day, Mimi remembers our account of that story. We hope she was as impacted by Craig as he was by her. Our family will never forget these young people, and we trust they have an added measure of understanding and love for the special needs people they encounter in their worlds today.

Chapter 11

The Balms of Gilead

Although teenagers and many other close friends had brought joy into Craig's life, he still experienced difficulties fitting completely into the church we attended. Small in stature, he had spent years with children younger than he, yet he needed a Sunday school class that would address his special requirements.

When Craig was thirteen Bill's employer transferred us to a city about two hours from the place Craig had always called home. With each transfer (five in all) we came to learn that something special was in store for Craig. After we had visited a lovely church in Centerville, Ohio, (transfer #1) we received a telephone call from the associate pastor informing us that he was very interested in starting a Sunday morning class for special needs persons. If we chose to continue attending the church, he assured us the class would start very soon.

Six weeks later I walked Craig to his own Sunday school class. It had not been an easy morning. It had taken me years to remember *not* to tell Craig to hurry and get dressed; unfortunately, those words threw him into his other speed, which was perilously close to *stop*. Somewhat frazzled by the time we arrived, I quietly explained this to Mrs. Neely, the teacher and the wife of the associate pastor. She reached for Craig and softly told me that whatever was needed to make his experience a success would be done, even if it meant tossing the lesson plans into the wastebasket. Then she said the most beautiful words to me, "Just go to your class and be ministered to." I walked away with tears in my eyes, humming that old hymn *There Is a Balm in Gilead* (1).

The Sunday school class created at *Washington Heights Baptist Church* that morning still exists, now serving some thirty adults each week. We are so thankful for this provision in our lives and in the lives of others it serves. Recently, the class celebrated its 25th anniversary, an event that was chronicled in a newsletter from *Shepherds Home and School*, a home for mentally challenged adults in Wisconsin. It was in that church and the previous church in Lima that Craig, during a Sunday evening service, stepped to the microphone and softly recited the names of all the books of the Bible, from Genesis to Revelation. The rote memory of these children is a gift that can be used in many ways. Craig had learned the books slowly and carefully, one at a time. Now, when he opens his Bible to follow a speaker, he knows how to locate the books.

Two years later (transfer #2) we were in another city searching for a church that would meet both our sons' needs. Our search was somewhat more extensive this time. After attending one church, a gentleman visited us in our home and kindly suggested that we find another one because he realized that the acceptance of special needs persons in his church was negligible.

And so our search continued. We finally settled at *Evangel Baptist Church* in Boardman, Ohio, where we felt a warm welcome. This time, however, a special needs class neither existed nor was formed. Instead Craig was mainstreamed with the fifth grade boys' class under the leadership of our friend and Bill's co-worker, Jerry. Jerry attended every special Olympic event in which Craig participated and included him with the other junior boys in day-long hikes and excursions. Craig was one of the boys, and this thrilled both him and us (inclusion at its best). And wonder of wonders, this qualified Craig for participation in the boys' and girls' Junior Choir. Craig was assigned his robe and collar and began attending rehearsals. He stood in the front row, proudly making his joyful noise along with the other singers who sang in tune and welcomed him with open arms.

Early one Easter morning Craig met with the Junior Choir members at the local mall to sing for a sunrise service. Bill and I took our places several rows from the choir, anticipating a beautiful service along with the other five hundred persons in attendance. Suddenly the choir director got our attention and motioned that Craig was ill. In fact, he was lying on the cold marble floor in a faint. Quickly, we made our way over to him, saw that he was awake, and covered him as he lay because the service was underway.

Little did we realize that his enthusiastic participation was not to be snuffed out by a mere fainting episode. When the choir kids assembled in their places and the introduction for their first number began, Craig jumped up, walked past the director (patting him on the shoulder), and took his place. The children simply stepped aside one-half step and gave him his front-row place. His face was white and his skin clammy, but his determination was undaunted; he made it through the two numbers without further mishap.

The next morning we placed a call to the doctor that had been treating him for hypothyroidism. He admitted Craig to Children's Hospital in Columbus, Ohio, and ran tests for a week, certain that the diagnosis would be juvenile onset sugar diabetes. But the doctor did not count on a choir of children in Boardman, Ohio, who were praying for their buddy. When the tests came back inconclusive, the choir kids were pleased, but not surprised. God had answered their prayers.

Our third transfer took us across the state of Ohio, where Craig joined an existing Sunday morning class for special needs persons in which he received sound Biblical instruction and enjoyed numerous social outings. The next transfer took us out of Ohio for the first time in our lives, to Virginia Beach where Craig took his place in an established Sunday school class taught by two dedicated men, Don and Jack. These men have worked selflessly and tirelessly for years, providing Biblical education at an understandable level for these dear adults.

Richmond, Virginia, became our last move. Craig attends a Special Persons Sunday school class at *Bon Air Baptist*, which offers a wonderfully balanced program of worship, Bible instruction, parties, picnics, hayrides, etc. He has many friends there and makes his way around the large church comfortably. On Sunday mornings Craig's feet are the first to hit the floor in our house, and he is dressed and ready to leave long before it's time to go. After several checks of the clock, pacing around the back door, and anxiously ushering us out the door, he scrambles into the car, excited to arrive at his own class early enough to have a cup of coffee with sugar.

Teaching techniques implemented in these classes often include first-person presentations of Bible stories by both the teaching staff and the students. It is not unusual for me to drop in on Craig's class and find him wearing a robe and a turban. At *Bon Air*, the Special Needs Class presented their portrayal of the nativity scene during a church-wide Christmas program recently. Dressed in full regalia of Bible costumes, they proudly made their way onstage to the manger to set up the tableau. Never mind that Mary was wearing tennis shoes, and that one of the Magi was so excited and pleased he could not stop grinning from ear to ear, nor that one of the shepherds tripped on his robe and required assistance moving up the steps. This was their very own telling of the greatest story ever told, and each and every person in the congregation was keenly aware just how much this portrayal meant to these special adults.

We have been blessed as the Lord has provided for Craig's spiritual development in every situation. The balms of Gilead just keep coming. So many wonderful people have impacted Craig's life; we trust that he, in turn, has exhibited God's love and has left his mark on them.

Chapter 12

The Most Important Event of My Life

"The most important event of my life is going to see my brother participate in Special Olympics. I like to see him run against his opponents and throw the softball.

He usually doesn't win, but when we congratulate him, he hugs us. To us he didn't win, but to him, just running or throwing the softball makes him a winner.

Most of the time I go down and take pictures of him and he gives me a big, goofy smile! I take pictures of him running or at the winners' table and of the crowd rooting for Craig.

After it's over, Craig brings home all the medals he won and hangs them on his bulletin board and talks about his day at Special Olympics."

—Kerry Sampson, age 12

In this fast-paced world of competition, pressure and tension, there is nothing more therapeutic than spending a day at a Special Olympics contest. Opening night brings hundreds of proud and excited contestants, some in wheelchairs, others walking with canes. They pour into the stands along with their dedicated trainers to begin a two-day schedule of athletic competitions.

Their motto: "Let me win, but if I cannot win, let me be brave in the attempt" (and if there is a parent there with dry eyes, he or she is the exception!). It actually means: *I'd like to win, but if you should fall, or if your shoestring should come undone, I will stop and help you.* Only then will the contest resume.

Time and again we see these special friends who have trained together halt a race to assist a fallen comrade. And across this country on the evening newscast, heartwarming pictures are shown of their unique brand of sportsmanship—their special brand of competition. How could we not learn from them?

When Eunice Kennedy Shriver, founder of Special Olympics, opened the first-ever International Special Olympics Summer Games on July 20, 1968, she spoke these words to the 1,000 athletes in attendance:

> "In ancient Rome, the gladiators went into the arena with these words on their lips: 'Let me win, but if I cannot win, let me be brave in the attempt.'
>
> "Today, all of you young athletes are in the arena. Many of you will win, but even more important, I know you will be brave, and bring credit to your parents and to your country. Let us begin the Olympics. Thank you" (1).

High-fives, handshakes and hugs abound at these events. Often, athletes from local colleges attend these events, milling around the crowd, exclaiming over newly won medals and autographing programs. When Kerry was in high school, he was already over six feet tall, and was often mistaken for one of the celebrities. Consequently, he spent the day signing, congratulating and hugging–and no one was the wiser.

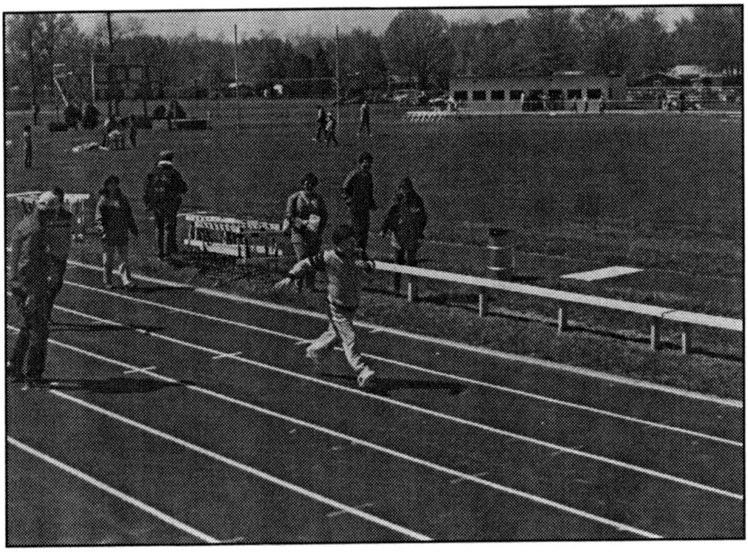

Craig heads for the finish line

During our years in Ohio, state Special Olympic competitions were held on the football field at O.S.U. For our two sons who are avid Ohio State football fans, spending two days on the campus of Ohio State, walking the same turf that the famed O.S.U. players and band performed was absolutely awesome.

One Sunday evening our family returned home after a weekend at Special Olympics just in time to attend Sunday evening church services. In one of his less humble moments, Craig sat in the pew proudly wearing two gold medals around his neck. Either Craig's beaming smile or the gold medals attracted the attention of the pastor, and from the pulpit he asked Craig how far he had thrown the softball to win his medal. The answer: "Real far!"

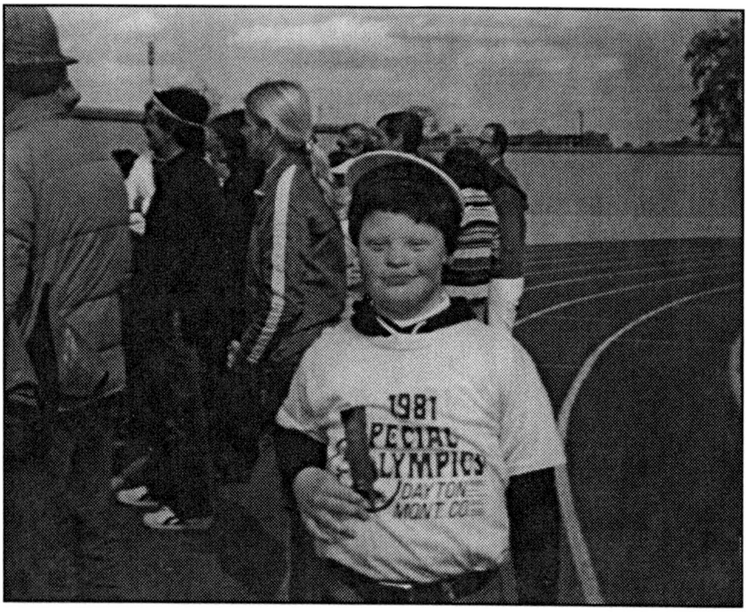

Craig proudly displays his blue ribbon

One comes away from these sporting events a changed person with a new perception of what is *really* important in life.

Chapter 13

R-E-T-A-R-D!

"R-E-T-A-R-D!" The quietness of the afternoon was shattered by the cruel name-calling. Stepping off the school bus, Craig was oblivious to the fact that the deprecation had been directed at him. However, his daddy, working in the garage, had overheard and was stunned.

Taking his son by the hand, Bill proceeded down the street to confront the offender. The guilty teenager had bolted for the safety of his room, but his friend consented to get him while Craig and his Dad waited in the driveway. Moments later the lad emerged, chagrined and shaken, apologizing profusely.

Bill is seldom ruffled and has a soft spot for teenagers. He realized this young man was acting out of ignorance and lack of understanding. After introducing the two boys (his name was Craig, too), Bill assured the teen that he had no intentions of making an issue of the episode. Rather he explained that although Craig is mentally challenged, he is not all that different from others kids as far as his interests in sports, music, etc. Our Craig, who was warmly smiling at his new friend all this time, offered his hand. The combination of two friendly faces was just too much for the young man; he apologized again and accepted Craig's proffered hand. Bill invited him to stop over anytime and get better acquainted with Craig.

An hour later, the lad was back saying, "That was a rotten thing to say; I'm really sorry!"

This event took place shortly after our family's first transfer to Centerville, Ohio. Craig had left his familiar surroundings, the friends and neighbors who knew and accepted him. Would he be able to cope with all the changes? He was again attending a segregated school for the developmentally delayed, riding the little yellow school bus for many miles each day. We wanted Craig to attend school in the district in which we lived. Public Law 94-142 (1) had been passed five years earlier. This law entitled special needs students to be placed in much less restrictive situations than the segregated schools could provide. Even a contained classroom located in a regular school would open up new opportunities for Craig to mingle occasionally with regular students, learning from them while having his own teachers and curriculum. Instead of learning survival techniques only in language and math, he could advance on an individual basis, removing the ceiling from his learning experience. Craig was not a high functioning student, but we knew he could do better. We were interested.

About this time we were contacted by some parents within the Centerville school district, inquiring about our interest in cooperating with a movement to get special classes established in their local schools to provide the integration we desired. At that time these were pilot programs, both innovative and controversial. We entered into their plans enthusiastically, yet cautiously. In the beginning two outstanding teachers were hired to teach two classes; one of them held multiple degrees—special education, physical therapy and speech therapy. The entire school and staff had been well prepared to accept these students by the use of a traveling puppet show entitled, New Kids on the Block (not the musicians!). In this presentation various handicaps were carefully explained, and students, using blindfolds, crutches, even cotton in the mouth to depict the obstacles faced by children with cerebral palsy, learned that these were just regular kids who coped with some unique problems.

Craig could now be mainstreamed for certain classes, and other selected regular students cooperated in the program in what was termed reverse mainstreaming. (We have watched the terms and acronyms change with regularity over the years. Inclusion is one of today's widely-used terms).

For a few months Craig was a participant of this program. Then we were transferred to Poland, Ohio. His academic skills had increased remarkably—going from recognizing a few survival words (stop, go, men, women, etc.) to reading on a primary level and learning to use a calculator for his math needs. We were sorry to have to leave, but were determined to stay the course after we moved.

About that time Craig went through some hormonal/behavioral changes (thirteen years of age, you know). Suddenly his behavior and language were affected; we were heartsick and appalled. I consulted with a psychologist who was experienced in dealing with special needs adults. One session with him and I came home with a notebook filled with instructions, including words I needed to use when approaching Craig. We felt we should keep him out of school until his behavior improved, and we did so for a few days. After a short time, Nabila, his teacher, called and said they wanted him back. She said they would deal with whatever came up, she understood our situation fully, and I was to bring Craig back, along with a sack of cookies for him to distribute to his classmates. The teachers would take it from there (another Balm of Gilead). When Craig arrived at school the next day, the entire class, along with all the teachers and students involved, stopped what they were doing and applauded his return. Craig was received warmly and the crisis began to pass. The expertise and support of his teachers at Centerville was absolutely amazing.

Most heartwarming of all was the story we heard two years after we had moved. By that time many of the regular students had become involved with the special needs class, using the buddy system, or reverse mainstreaming. They loved it. Due to some restructuring of the school system, the school board had determined the special needs class must be pulled out of that school and moved elsewhere. Their buddies were heartbroken. An emotional school board meeting was held, allowing the public to vent their views. Parents of regular students testified to the maturity this experience had brought to their children and requested reconsideration by the school board. The evening news relayed the essential content of this meeting, along with tearful parents and children. The outcome? The class for special needs stayed. Somehow, I wasn't surprised. God is an awesome God!

"...Inasmuch as ye have done it unto one of the least of these my brethren, ye have done it unto me" (2).

Chapter 14

Educational Pioneering

The success of the innovative, progressive educational program at Centerville Schools forever altered our thinking regarding methods of teaching the developmentally delayed students. No longer were we willing to place Craig in the safe, yet restrictive environment of the schools that accommodate only special needs students—the segregated schools. While Craig was not high functioning, we had witnessed many children who were lower functioning than he profit tremendously from being placed in a less restrictive environment. They learned to drop certain inappropriate behaviors that were, sad to say, often the hallmark of persons with mental handicaps. Attention was given to hygiene, hairstyles, up-to-date clothing, and elimination of speech and movements that were different from other students. In addition the instructors began focusing on academics that would serve them well the rest of their lives. Whether or not to choose this type of classroom setting was, and still is, a decision that must be individually made by parents, and I respect all who carefully think their way through this choice. But they should have that choice. Our eyes had been opened, and we were now equipped with information and contacts in the state in which we lived. We realized that we had to spearhead that drive in our new community.

Our next transfer (#2) took us to the opposite corner of the same state, Poland, Ohio, and we chose to move into a fairly small school district that was highly rated academically out of consideration for Kerry. However, the district, by comparison to the one we had left, was much smaller, which made money an issue (isn't it always?). While this school had performed well on the basics, they did not have the progressive vision of the one we'd left. The school administration could not understand why we refused to place Craig in the segregated school there; they had nothing else to offer. Consequently Craig was tutored at home for a year, then we agreed to allow him to be transported to a special needs class housed in a junior high school in an adjoining county.

Meanwhile Bill and I continued our battle for the local school to provide better programs for the developmentally disadvantaged. We participated in a seven-state meeting in Minnesota, outlining ideas on both educational and vocational programs, and we spoke at Kent State University in northeastern Ohio, explaining our position to a several-county task force comprised of approximately two hundred teachers, therapists and administrators. I also attended and participated in countless forums in an effort to gain support and enlighten parents of their rights.

The national economy was going through a decline, and the city nearby was particularly affected due to recent closing of steel mills. Schools did not have extra dollars to spend, and people were concerned with their jobs; education was not the top priority. Change and modification were difficult for them to cope with at that time, and we understood. Still we knew that with careful planning and prudent expenditure of available state funding, the educational program for the mentally and developmentally challenged could be vastly improved. So we persisted. We persisted to the point that the superintendent of the local school in which we lived stated aloud that he wished we would move to another school district!

Finally after contacting the Ohio State Board of Education and clarifying our legal position, we met with state board representatives and the local school administrator. The state board fully backed us, advising the school administrator that he could set up what we wanted for less than his legal fees would be. As a result of this meeting, the Poland Schools acquiesced to our request.

This process moved *very* slowly, and we had to settle for at-home tutoring and transporting Craig to another county in the meantime. The upside to having Craig home 24/7 was that I had opportunities to instruct him in self-skills. Sometimes I got myself into trouble, such as the day I decided to train him to go into a lockdown whenever I needed to run an errand. Carefully and thoroughly we went over the business of locking all outside doors and allowing the answering machine to take any calls. This would free me to occasionally run a twenty-minute errand. Two days into our training program, I decided to give Craig a test. Lurking in the street one block away, I witnessed Craig's return from school, gave him time to execute his lockdown, then drove back to the house, opened the garage door with the remote and parked the car in the garage. When I attempted to enter the house through the garage door, I discovered my mistake. I had no house key with me because I always used that handy little remote, and everything was locked tightly. For forty-five minutes I intermittently rang the doorbell and called to Craig, explaining in very loud tones that I was his mother and he could now unlock the door. For a while he stood inside the foyer and actually talked to me, but would not unlock the door. Finally Craig granted me admittance through the front door. I was chagrined, relieved, proud, and embarrassed all at once, because the neighbors had taken great delight in the unfolding drama at our house.

Fortunately progress was made on the schooling issues, and local parents were becoming enthusiastic! You guessed it; we were transferred once more. My consolation came in the form of phone calls and notes sent by grateful parents as the new educational program unfolded.

Chapter 15

The Turning Point

The addresses presented by Bill and me on February 11, 1983, at Kent State University in northeastern Ohio clearly portray the educational battles regarding special education in Ohio some twenty-three years ago. Hopefully this controversy now is settled both in Ohio and in our country as a whole. You will note as you read these presentations that the terms have changed—MR, SMI, etc.—but the premises remain the same. In order to swing the educational thinking in our direction, we had to present a strong case for desegregation of special needs students. Bill presented first as follows:

"In the years Joyce and I have been married, we have been blessed with two very special sons—Craig, a sixteen-year-old with Down syndrome and Kerry, a thirteen-year-old with lots of energy. We would like to share with you today a little of Craig's educational background as well as our conviction and commitment to a public school environment for MR (Mentally Retarded) students.

Craig became a part of a segregated system at the age of eighteen months and at age fourteen we made the decision to withdraw him from the segregated school and enroll him in an SMI (Severely Mentally Impaired) program in the public school.

SMI, mainstreaming, reverse mainstreaming, a non-segregated educational approach for Craig—all these are terms and ideas we were aware of, but never pursued. Why? Why would two parents who were convinced Craig's educational needs were not being met be so long in addressing this situation?

We tried! For several years we felt Craig had the ability to read and perform simple math. However, we had neither the education nor the training to adequately teach Craig the academic skills he desperately needed, and the school simply was not getting this accomplished. We had attended board meetings and requested reading programs—without success. To a certain degree Craig's social needs were being met in school, but we felt socialization was primarily our responsibility. Every person, normal or MR, needs more than social graces. Joyce will address this in a few moments.

There are a couple of reasons the educational process for Craig did not materialize earlier, in particular from the time of the passage of Public Law 94-142 (which insured that each child with disabilities would be schooled in the least restrictive environment). The reasons are *fear* and *work*!

Fear on the part of public schools to institute innovative programs such as the SMI concept. How do we teach normal children to accept the MR children? How do we get our teachers to implement such a program and accept a "retarded kid" for mainstreaming? Let *them* stay in a school where they belong with others of their kind was the prevailing attitude. In addition, parents of normal children resisted. Sometimes we felt that others thought retardation was a communicable disease. It isn't! Further, *fear* was and still is in the minds of parents of MR children. The last thing we want is for our child to be made fun of and kidded about something he cannot control.

This is where the *work* comes in. How does change begin and where does it start? You must understand here that these are my ideas as a parent; as educators you may disagree, but I'll share them anyway. It seems to me that county offices are the base; they have a tremendous responsibility to inform local schools of their responsibility and work with them in producing a quality program. A program, just because *we have to*, will not be successful. There is a need to work with parents to enlighten and inform them of the availability of alternative education for their children. This is not accomplished with one or two meetings. Many questions arise because each parent is vitally concerned as to how mental and physical problems will be addressed. *Work* on the part of public school teachers and staff to prepare their normal students for kids who are different. This is a sizable undertaking but I can tell you it is phenomenally rewarding!

A job transfer took us to Centerville, Ohio in 1979 and two school terms in a segregated system for our son, Craig. The spring of 1980 was the beginning of a dramatic change for him. We had received a letter requesting us to attend a parents' meeting with Centerville's Pupil Services Coordinator to discuss the possibility of starting an SMI program in the Centerville Schools. I attended that meeting with the *fear* I spoke about earlier, i.e. students will make fun of Craig. I even voiced my concern and stated I was not sure we were willing to cooperate. I should have waited. Mr. Browning had done his homework well and he asked other parents to share with us the benefits of public school education. As the months and meetings passed, the excitement grew. We saw all the *fears* and *work* I described earlier translate to action, and in the fall of 1981 Centerville Schools inaugurated their (our) SMI program. Craig was in the program for twelve weeks, and I don't have time to tell of the progress made.

Twelve weeks into his program another transfer occurred—this time, Poland, Ohio. I would like to tell you the result here was as positive as before, but it was not. Remember *Fear* and *Work?* Neither the county nor the local school district shared our enthusiasm for SMI classes. We were firmly committed to public education, so Craig was not enrolled in a segregated school here. After a five-week delay, Craig began private at-home tutoring for the duration of the 1981-82 school term.

Unfortunately numerous meetings and phone calls did not result in an SMI program in our school district. It was not until late summer last year that we were able to begin serious negotiations with the Superintendent of Schools in Poland. At a meeting with Drs. Gross and Saylor of the State Department of Education and the Superintendent, we were able to amicably work out an agreement for schooling that would be beneficial to Craig. The result was Craig's enrollment in a very progressive SMI unit at Lincoln School in Niles, with transportation provided.

I would like my wife, Joyce, to share with you the benefits Craig derived from the SMI program, both in Centerville and Niles."

"Prior to the fall opening of the original SMI classes in Centerville, a summer program was implemented in order that the teaching staff and coordinators could observe our children and become acquainted with each one and his or her unique needs. This program accomplished various things such as introducing the children to one another, the staff and the school, and familiarizing them with the classroom setting. With the first day of school in August came the removal of a significant barrier for our children—the banishment of segregated education. To us segregation in any form is less than desirable. Most of our children had been a part of a lifestyle of integration; they were accustomed to living, shopping, going to church, ballgames, etc., in their communities. Now they could go to school with their peers instead of riding a bus as long as ninety minutes each way to a county-based, segregated school. We believe that education in the least restrictive environment is impossible to attain in a segregated school.

It is thrilling to share with you the progress evidenced by Craig in the SMI environment. In Centerville's SMI program, expectations for each child ran higher than the child had ever previously known—no limits were set. Each child was permitted and encouraged to *try*, expected to *work* and even allowed the occasional lesson of failure. The instructors recognized that occasional failure does not destroy a handicapped child. After all everyone in life fails at something; many of us learn much in those situations. The important thing is to have some successes, too, in order to provide a balance.

As part of their physical therapy program, a swimming program was arranged for the SMI students and they were expected to learn to swim and become water-safe—which they did. No longer was Craig permitted to simply don his swimsuit and blow bubbles in the water as he had done for years. At first this resulted in reluctance on his part— "forgetting" his swimsuit on Thursdays, and informing mother that "swimming has been cancelled." But when he began to experience success, his attitude changed rapidly! Today, nearly all of those Centerville students have learned to swim.

No longer acceptable were forms of inappropriate behavior, too often the earmark of MR children. Discourtesies, inappropriate language, and excessive affection simply were not permitted in order for mainstreaming to be a successful venture. With the correction of these behaviors and the effect of role modeling of regular school children, an incredible normalization of our children occurred. One could walk into the SMI classrooms at any given time and observe sixteen students tending to task, many working independently, but all working quietly and diligently. On the walls hung each child's IEP, posted there for easy referral, with reports going home at least weekly to apprise parents of progress made and improvements needed.

One of the important factors that contribute greatly to the success of the SMI unit in a least restrictive setting is peer role modeling. Normal children surrounded Craig and his classmates. Centerville utilized the buddy system, or reverse mainstreaming, which brought a steady flow of non-handicapped students into the units. Some SMI students left the units to attend regular classes for music, art, physical education, library, math, reading and social studies at first and second grade levels. Access to all those programs was determined by the readiness of each MR student to be mainstreamed. Group assemblies, puppet shows, movies and flag ceremonies were available to all handicapped students. Our children were stretched and enriched by these close contacts with the non-handicapped; conversely, normal children took great pride from interaction with ours. I have talked with parents who were glowing with the satisfaction their children received from working with ours as peer tutors. "Knowledge our children could have never acquired from a textbook," was a common parental remark. And parents went on record to state they wanted the program for the handicapped in the public schools to continue. These comments, I might add, were made near the close of the first year of SMI classes at Centerville and were a complete reversal of parents' earlier attitudes!

Indeed, as time went on, the effect of our children was evidenced upon their peers and teachers as well. Fear changed to acceptance, acceptance to sensitivity and caring and sharing in our children's growth. One 4-5th grade teacher, in particular, tremendously influenced her students to reach out to ours. This changing attitude soon reached into the community as well. Craig was named an honorary member of his brother's soccer team that fall (due in part to his faithful attendance and very vocal support at the games), and was presented a team shirt complete with SAMPSON lettered across the back. Later when the team won runner-up trophies, he was again included, and that trophy sits front and center on his dresser to this day!

During the twelve weeks Craig was involved in Centerville's unit, we observed a sizable improvement in his social behavior and maturity level as well. He desired to be more independent in self-help skills such as bathing, dressing, eating, and selecting clothes. He became more aware of those around him and fit himself in with groups of children easily. My husband and I were directors of a large junior high church group at that time and Craig was very comfortable interacting with them.

But now I get to the thrilling part of Craig's story—academics! To many sixteen-year olds, academics are something less than thrilling. But to Craig, they are the beginning of a whole new dimension in his life.

For six or seven years I had attempted to get more emphasis on academics at his school. As psychologists would interview Craig and me and subsequently report, they would say, "Mother requests more time spent on reading, math and handwriting." We wanted his time at school to be spent on learning these skills. *We* were willing to provide bowling, parties, field trips, etc., to stimulate him socially. But our son was en route or at school many hours per day, and he came home tired and hungry and in no mood to work at reading skills. In addition I am not an educator—I do not possess the training to work with him—yet as I experimented and saw the potential he had (a retentive memory and an ear for phonics), I became even more convinced he could learn to read books at least on a primary level. The first segregated school did not even own or implement a school-wide reading curriculum; to read or not to read was left to the discretion of the teacher (who may have the same child for up to three years), most of whom opted for the teaching of some 50 survival words only. The second segregated school did have a *Distar* reading curriculum, but they informed us that they did not have enough aides to do any individual teaching.

When I approached the Centerville teaching staff about our goals, they were very encouraging and supportive. To make a long story short, Craig made abounding progress in those twelve weeks, not only in reading but in basic math skills as well. His handwriting became much more legible even though fine and gross motor skills are still his greatest weak points.

November 26th, 1981, our moving van left Centerville, delivering us to Poland School District in Mahoning County, Ohio. Before accepting this transfer with GMAC, my husband had received information by phone that two SMI classes were available in Mahoning County. We were to discover later that these classes served non-ambulatory residents of a local nursing home. This, obviously, was not an appropriate placement for our son.

After much deliberation, spanning the months of October through December, we finally agreed to at-home tutoring, two hours a day, with no related services for the duration of the school year, with the promise of SMI classes here by the fall of 1982.

Within six weeks Craig was doing simple math and reading simple sentences. There would be no question about his comprehension if you were to hear him read. He is very pleased with himself and his newly acquired skills. (His tutor remarked that Craig had been ready to read for a long time.) Today this type education continues for him in a well-run SMI class in Niles, where Craig is mainstreamed whenever possible with sixth graders.

Academic skills, maturity growth, improved social skills, acceptance by the community—all are vital ingredients in the total development of persons with disabilities and very significant reasons for the Sampsons' continued belief in educating the handicapped in public schools, the least restrictive setting. We have the advantage of comparison, and we clearly see that the SMI placement benefits our son. I am acquainted with many parents of lower-functioning children than Craig who feel as strongly as we do. We as parents know our kids better than any other person on earth. We live and breathe with them every day. We see their reactions and non-reactions, their abilities and disabilities. We can tell when they are putting forth all their possible effort or just playing for attention. We parents see and feel our child's developments each and every day. The responsibility falls upon us to be their advocates, to have the courage and assertiveness to speak for their needs.

Our commitment to advocacy for Craig was made years ago, in the fall of 1966, to be exact—when Craig was born. We are a Christian family; our home is committed to Christ and His precepts. Shortly after Craig's birth we came to grips with his retardation and vowed to do our utmost to insure that he developed his fullest potential in every way. Long ago we stopped struggling with the disappointment and bitterness and realized the value of this very special gift from God. Carrying out this vow has meant being strong in our position (even arbitrary at times); it has meant having to let him *go* to *grow* when as a mother, I wanted to shield and over-protect. But a vow is not to be taken lightly, and God has even supplied the pioneer spirit!

We *are* pioneering in this corner of the state of Ohio. As a special education administrator in Centerville challenged educators and parents last March with these words, so we, in closing, similarly challenge you.

> We must be daring and innovative. If we protect our children from society by keeping them in a closed program for twenty-two years, we can hardly expect the rest of the world to welcome this different, even strange creature with open arms when they have never met him. It is not enough to take our children to the store, to the zoo, to the movies. The public has to have more involvement than a casual, visual passing. They have to get to know these children and to be involved on a daily basis with them. I am not protecting my child by keeping him separate. You are not protecting him.

We are just delaying the inevitable, the movement back into the community, unless we are willing to accept the old barren, walled-in institutions of the past. I am not. Many parents of young handicapped children are not, and the numbers are growing. Let's avoid the costs of court suits and lengthy angry hostility and spend the time and money on educating children. Let's allow all children a true public school education. Let's allow our child and others like him to have the challenge of high expectations and peer models to encourage them to do their best" (1).

Chapter 16

It's All About Friends!

Our journeys from city to city may sound daunting to some who have never experienced a move or a transfer. True, it is not easy to pack up your belongings, find a home and start anew in a strange city. But it can also be challenging, adventurous and exciting! We chose to view it in that way. Looking back and remembering all the people we have come to know, even for a short time, we have concluded that we would not trade our journey for anything.

In every city friendships were formed, many of which are still active. Other friends we no longer hear from on a regular basis, but their impact on our lives is lasting. During our Lima, Ohio days, we enjoyed the friendship of Paul, Margene, and their daughters, Michelle and Melanie, with whom we celebrated our children's birthdays, vacationed together, and spent hours at the local swim club together. We have also been blessed with dear friends—the Snyders, Brants, and Nelsons (Yoakams)—who have remained close through every move we made. Our children grew up with these friends, we vacationed with them, attended church together, and we still find a way to spend a weekend together here and there. They are always welcome in our home—wherever it is!

During Craig's growing-up years, our friends' children were his buddies.

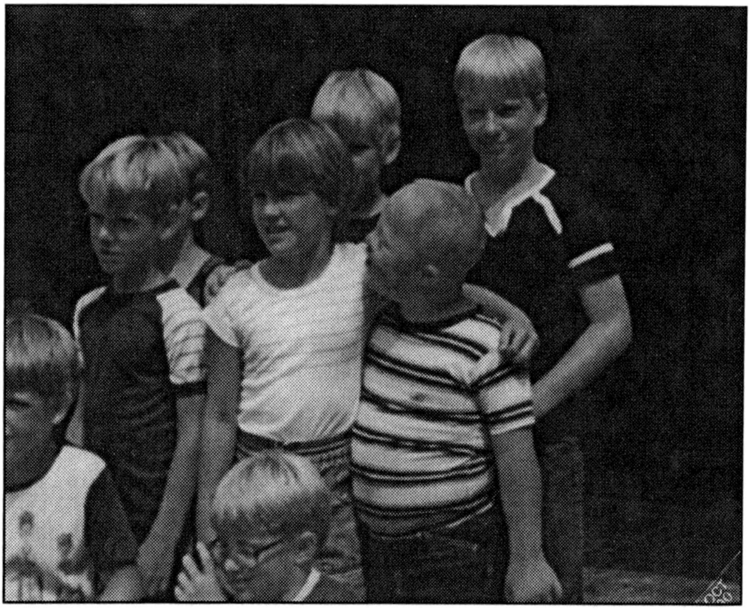

Craig with arms around his friends

When our four families vacationed together in Pennyroyal State Park, Kentucky (pronounced Pennyrile), Craig spent the week in the thick of things, trying desperately to keep up with all the activities.

Pennyroyal State Park borders on a lake with fishing, swimming, camping, and golfing offered, and the younger set of children loved to grab fishing poles, set out for the bridge and try their luck. One afternoon the children returned after a few minutes and went on to some other activity. In the meantime Craig-come-lately set out for the bridge to find them, did not locate them at the fishing place, and continued on his own, walking over dangerous rocky trails clear around the lake.

Our entire group was frantically searching for him, growing more and more panicky by the moment. Mike ran all the way around the lake, calling for Craig. He did not locate him, but he did discover a folded piece of paper, which we called Craig's *shake*, lying on the path, a testament to the fact that Craig had, indeed, made his way around those trails.

We learned later that a couple in a Volkswagen picked up Craig when he emerged from the path on the other side of the lake. This kind couple took him to the campsite where the chef of the lodge's dining room recognized Craig, loaded him into his vehicle and drove back to the lodge site, horn blaring. By this time local search teams, even a lake dredging team, had assembled to assist in the hunt.

They explained the bridge Craig had crossed was narrow and treacherous, especially for one who was an unstable climber. Needless to say we were profoundly relieved and grateful—not

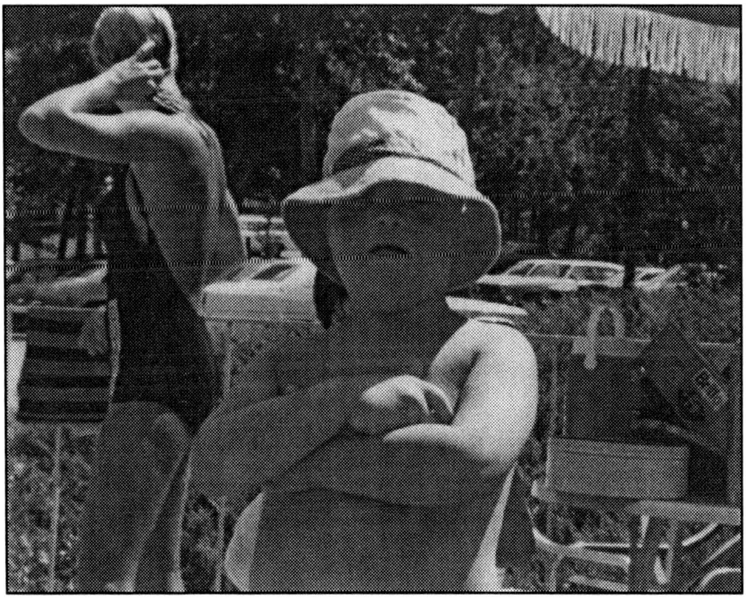

Craig at Pennyrile

to mention slightly hysterical! Craig, however, having enjoyed the attention and the noisy return, took the whole episode in stride.

Music has continued its impact in Craig's life, becoming almost an electronic friend. His huge library of tapes and CDs is in constant use and accompanies him whenever we take long road trips. Once—just once—I decided to set him up with earphones and tapes in the backseat of the car, thinking that Bill and I could enjoy a nice conversation while we traveled, instead of singing along with Craig's tapes of children's Christian music (which were great, but grew a wee bit tiresome after a while). About two miles down the road, we realized that we were now being treated to hearing only Craig's voice without the advantage of his back-up singers. The earphones went into retirement.

Craig's friends encompass all age groups; he's very much a people person. Former neighbors, Dave and Mary Jane, who have since moved to Florida, lure Craig (and us) regularly for visits. After spending a few days in their swimming pool and boating on the beautiful waters of the Gulf, Craig announced to them that he loved their lifestyle–"swimmin' and eatin' out!" When his friends are not physically surrounding him, he substitutes his crayons for them, drawing circles and roads on the floor of our family room around him, naming each crayon. On his 25th birthday he received 110 cards from family and friends from the five cities in which we had lived. The cards are his prized possessions; they reside in a big plastic box, and he spends each evening opening them up one-by-one, reading the verses and signatures. His delight in life is bringing a smile to the face of a friend.

Chapter 17

The Toledo Years–Badges, Lollipops and Wastebaskets

A near-blizzard was the prevailing weather when the moving van rolled out of Poland, Ohio. Our next destination across the state, Toledo, Ohio, shares the borders of Lake Erie with the state of Michigan. Temperatures hovered around zero when we finally checked into our motel around 1:30 a.m. The next morning we waited in our new, but empty house for the moving van to show up. It seemed the van's frozen motor refused to cooperate when attempts were made to start it (we'd had the same problem when the alarm had gone off). Two hours later the van arrived and the flurry of unpacking began.

Although winters were somewhat harsh, summers in Toledo were beautiful and we quickly settled into our new routine. This move brought us closer to our original home, only two hours away from Lima. Now we had access to our families and friends and we eagerly anticipated enjoyable times.

Craig was nineteen at this point, and his educational years were nearly over. During the summers he worked with a group assembled by Lucas County (yes!), painting the interior of an elementary school. The first year and a half we were there, Craig was transported (again) to a neighboring county for special education classes in an elementary school. However, he was elevated during the second year to a resource class at Whittier High School in Toledo, where he had the good fortune of being taught by Mrs. "O", Corrine Oliger, along with her able assistant, Mrs. Cole.

Craig's maturation during those two years was remarkable. The students were integrated into the school's classes and activities whenever feasible. In the resource classroom, they learned to prepare their own lunches, using portable equipment, and made many practical and functional field trips to improve their self-help and survival skills, all the while progressing well with their academics. They even started their own company, catering hors d'oeuvres for teachers' functions, having raised start-up funds by making and selling badges and chocolate lollipops to the student body. The feeling of independence achieved during those two years brought a huge measure of pride and self-confidence to Craig and his fellow students.

At home Craig lived out the training he was receiving at school. Craig and Kerry often served as waiters whenever Bill and I entertained. Once at a progressive dinner held at our house for adult church friends, the boys dressed in shirts and ties—and jams, colorful Bermuda shorts, with checkered towels draped carefully over their arms. Greeting our guests at the door brought startled looks to our guests' faces, but the boys enjoyed it immensely.

Soon Craig began looking around the house for ways to help me, assigning himself such tasks as setting and clearing the table, emptying wastebaskets, putting laundry away and cleaning his room. The pride that accompanied his new status at our house was quite apparent. Occasionally as I assembled a meal and worked around the house, I found that I had to share my space (all right, I often tripped over him). *Every* day he emptied *every* wastebasket, then set up a watch to see whether or not someone had the nerve to drop a piece of paper into one.

One morning I was leaning over my dressing table, applying make-up, when he charged into the room, brushed me aside and reached for the wastebasket. Although this had happened numerous times before, I lost patience this time. "Craig", I said, "There's absolutely nothing in that wastebasket!" He surveyed the emptiness of the wastebasket, replied, "Oops!" and promptly reached in front of me for a tissue which he deposited in the wastebasket and took off at full speed to empty it. Now a lot older and a little wiser, I have learned to choose my battles.

Much of Craig's time and focus during the Toledo years was spent with Kerry and his friends who came regularly to the house. Kerry was playing high school basketball, and Craig's attendance at his games was a real highlight. Even though Kerry was nearly three years younger, he was now the big brother and assumed a good share of protectiveness and responsibility towards his little brother. In fact Kerry stayed with Craig often, freeing Bill and me to go out, even overnight. From two little toddlers who had parallel-played together, through the reversal-of-roles years, they had emerged, still buddies. Kerry has been the perfect role model for Craig; we could not have asked for more, and we are grateful.

Chapter 18

Special Persons Mailing Service

The sunny beaches of Virginia were the location of our next-to-last transfer—our first experience living in the mid-south, in fact, our first move out of the state of Ohio. I mention this because we were greatly impacted by the move as we searched for educational/vocational training for Craig.

First of all we had to learn a new vocabulary. Any parents working with children who have disabilities know that the terms, initials and acronyms surrounding the delivery of services to the mentally challenged change rapidly. We also learned these terms vary from state to state. It took us some time to learn the structure and organization of the agencies that serve this special population in Virginia. Craig would have had one more year of school in Ohio. However, Virginia's deadline was different and we discovered that Craig had completed his schooling. The search was on for programs that would get him into the community around the stimulation of other people, and, of course, we wanted him placed in a vocational position.

Recreationally we had come to the right place. Virginia Beach is an exciting place in which to live; there are activities going on year-around, and the local recreational centers offer many programs for the special needs population. Craig met with his friends once a week to swim, once a week to bowl, and frequently to picnic together. He even took a course in living skills at the community college. He also participated in a program sponsored by the city, which took him from water parks to marine museums to sand sculpturing at the beach. He became acquainted with the area far more rapidly than we did, and began directing us around.

Vocationally we had to exercise patience. Just as we had not wanted Craig isolated in a special school during his educational years, we did not want him segregated in a large workshop for his working years. After a long wait, during which time he enjoyed many field trips, we finally placed him in a workshop, temporarily. (By this time he had already seen everything at the beach at least twice.) The workshop, located one mile from our home, was well operated, and Craig acquired some new skills, but I was on the lookout for something better.

One morning Craig was swimming at the Kempsville Recreation Center, when I noticed a gentleman there accompanying his daughter who also had Down syndrome. We struck up a conversation, and he told me of a small non-profit business he was starting in his home to provide work for his Jennifer and a couple of friends. It would be a mailing service—collating, stuffing, sealing and stamping envelopes. The plan was to grow the business to ten or twelve persons, and he invited us to consider it for Craig. His enthusiasm was contagious, and I, too, became excited about his plans. That is, until I discovered that the location was about a twenty-five minute drive from my home—a trip through a busy city which I would have to make twice daily. At the close of our conversation, I gave him Craig's and my names and phone numbers, written on a sewing pattern order form, the only piece of paper I had in my pocket. When I returned home and reflected upon my meeting a strange man and giving him my phone number, I could not believe what I had done. But when one meets Art Roy, he/she meets a man who is people-oriented, has a pleasant, positive outlook on life and a great sense of humor. I just knew Craig would integrate well into his plans—and that Bill would understand (he did).

For two years I continued to transport Craig to the workshop, wishing all the time for something better for him. When the city decided to close that facility and move the workshop miles away, I knew it was time to call Mr. Roy. Sometimes God has to make his plans pretty obvious to me.

One December morning Bill called Mr. Roy, identified himself and Craig, and asked if he had any openings in his growing business, now called Special Persons Mailing Service (SPMS). Before he could finish his question, Art said, "I've been waiting for you to call! I have your name and phone number right here in my desk drawer, expecting to hear from you someday soon."

An appointment was set up for a work evaluation, and Bill and I escorted an excited Craig for the first time to SPMS. I said excited, didn't I? When Craig gets excited or nervous, he becomes very quiet, even quieter than usual. Mr. Roy and his daughter were the only two working that morning, and he trained and observed Craig for a couple hours. Upon our return Shari had joined them, a petite young lady whose parents have been very actively involved in the business. Shari is as outgoing as Craig is shy. When Mr. Roy introduced Craig to Shari and announced that he was their newest employee, Shari looked directly at Craig and queried, "Do you like girls?" In his soft, low voice, Craig replied, "Yeah!" Grins and huge hugs were exchanged and Craig was *in*—both vocationally and socially.

Craig began working for SPMS shortly thereafter and loved it. The business had grown to accommodate ten young people who, like Craig, lived with their parents. Mr. Roy trained each of his employees, then painstakingly trained parents as well (sometimes this was the greater challenge). Being a non-profit organization the volunteer assistance of parents and friends was vital. Only the special needs persons were paid. Typically parents donated their time for a day each week.

These young people arrived on time each morning, ready to work. They raced each other in from the parking lot to the back door, and were ready and eager to begin work at the stroke of nine, if not before. This employment was a dream fulfilled for several of them who had had negative experiences with past employers. Tommy, a delightful, mannerly man who was fascinated with computers and with the beautiful paneled office belonging to the Norfolk naval base chaplain, had always dreamed of working either with the chaplain or in a similar office. One afternoon as we worked feverishly trying to make deadlines, someone loudly announced that Tommy had just left the mailing service and was walking toward the nearby bank, planning to land a job there (where they had paneled offices). Mr. Roy gave him a little space, then, realizing that Tommy meant business, started out after him. After a soft drink and a little conversation, Tommy returned to us, satisfied that *this* job truly fulfilled his dream—a dream that just needed a little adjustment.

We watched that wonderful little business expand, outgrow its rented building and be moved into a new facility. In May 1995, *People* magazine wrote a three-page feature article on SPMS, complete with pictures of our crew at work. The employees celebrated birthdays together, participated in recreational center activities, and enjoyed swim parties in the summer, Christmas parties in the winter. I cannot say enough about Art Roy, his wife, Floy, the Whittles who were instrumental in the start-up, Ed Hardin and other parents who have kept the business going and growing so these young adults could always have a place to work.

Occasionally we have returned to visit SPMS. Craig is always received with shouts of welcome and open arms. The last time we visited, Craig had packed his lunch, unnoticed by us, and charged out of the car and into the SPMS building in a flash.

We had intended to stay for a few minutes. Craig, with the encouragement of Mr. Roy, spent the day. Mr. Roy waved to us as we left; Craig did not even acknowledge that we had gone.

By this point in our lives, we were finally realizing the Lord was not going to duplicate our experiences from city-to-city. Rather He had something special in store for us with each move. He was teaching us to lean on Him. From the creation of the Shepherds Sunday school class in Centerville, Ohio, to inclusion in the junior boys Sunday school class and the Junior Choir in Poland, Ohio, to two other special needs classes in Toledo, Ohio, and Norfolk, Virginia, to Mrs. "O" and now this. He just kept on blessing and blessing.

Chapter 19

Grandparents and Polar Bears

September 23, 1966. When he walked into the hospital room, he simply gathered his little girl into his arms and hugged her without a word. My usually undemonstrative father had come home from a hard day's work, showered and rushed to the hospital to console his daughter after hearing the news surrounding Craig's birth.

My dad was an identical twin, raised during hard times and educated during the depression years. His early life had not been easy; he had learned out of necessity a variety of hands-on skills. He could fix anything. And he wanted to fix the dilemma that now faced his daughter and son-in-law. But it wasn't to be.

The role my father quickly assumed was to encourage us and support our efforts. During Craig's first years, my dad was often at a loss about how to relate to him. He held him, and sang to him, and often picked him up, later, from school, but it was difficult for him to really understand and relate to Craig, one-on-one. When Kerry arrived dad saw his chance to effectively assist us by spending time with *him*—the *other* child who often gets overlooked in a family where a special needs child exists. Dad poured himself into Kerry's life, and a mutual love and respect developed that exists today, some eight years after dad's death. While he taught Kerry many of the same skills he possessed, more importantly he established within our son the assurance and confidence that Grampy was there for him. His impact will be felt for the duration of Kerry's life.

On the other hand my mother quickly took matters into her own hands and began to assist me. Carefully she watched me sing-and-spoon food into Craig's mouth. Then, when she was sure she had the hang of it, she was ready to shoo me away to attend support meetings and grocery shop. An at-home wife, she was available to Craig-sit and did so willingly. She was extremely sensitive to my emotional needs, driving to my house once a week for several years to watch the boys while I got my hair done or shopped. Many times, she would check our church bulletin to see what meetings I should be attending, then offer to Craig-sit. Their bond was tight; when she became ill with breast cancer, Craig just *knew* something was terribly wrong. During her illnesses Craig was the only one who could get her a glass of water and tuck her in *just right.* She battled breast cancer, her second round, for eight years, willing herself to live because Craig needed her (and so did I!). Needless to say her home-going left a huge void. Craig remained in anger for months, even years. He could not understand why his grandmother would leave him.

Craig was one of fourteen grandchildren on Bill's mother's side. A seamstress at a brace and limb shop, she worked full-time, yet she did an amazing job of spending time with each of her beloved grandchildren.

When Craig spent time with her, she would play games and make use of his rote memory, teaching him Bible verses. After she retired she would come for visits wherever we were, and spend several days–a huge highlight for Craig and us. She passed away after a long illness and all the grandchildren were asked to be pallbearers at her memorial service, including Craig. He had not the slightest idea what a pallbearer was and did not take kindly to

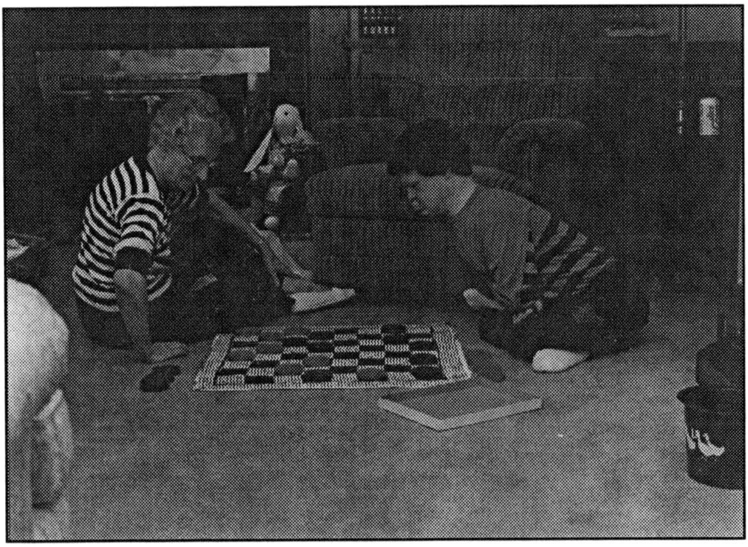

Craig with Grandma

funerals. After some cajoling and encouragement, plus a promise that he could walk alongside his cousin, Todd, and be shown what to do, he consented to do this for his grandmother.

In the car on the way home the conversation went like this:

"Dad, do you know what I did for my grandmother at her fo'neral today?"

"No, son, what did you do?"

"I was a polar bear!"

Chapter 20

Repeat and Recap

With lots of good-byes and hugs, Craig and I drove away from the Special Persons Mailing Service—one of the most difficult things I have ever done. The moving van was transporting us to Richmond, Virginia, our final move before Bill's retirement from GMAC. Craig's employment in Richmond in the ten years we have lived here has been varied, yet steady, thanks to his case manager, Dan, and Chesterfield Employment Services. However, SPMS will always be the highlight of his employment days and he often relives his experiences and mentions the friends with whom he worked. We pray that business will continue to flourish.

Although the relocations have been challenging and sometimes difficult, they have brought us together as a family and increased our dependence upon the Lord. Our outlooks were broadened by the exposure to new things—cities, schools, cultures, food, neighbors, friends, and churches. Craig, who loved the comfort of order and routine, was compelled to learn to adjust frequently to new surroundings and schedules. From a child who had often refused to leave his comfort zone, he has matured to an enthusiastic "Can I go?" whenever he sniffs new plans afoot. Most of all we cherish the people who have come into his life, all of whom left a positive impact. He has been so blessed with caring people. Aunts, uncles, cousins, neighbors, church friends and family friends have gone out of their way repeatedly to show their love and acceptance.

Having mastered the rudiments of lockdown, Craig enjoys a little time alone in the house while his Mom and Dad run an errand or two. He is very responsible regarding care of the house, even to rearranging furniture and smaller items to satisfy his own taste. Our former neighbors, Peggy and Jerry, kept a watchful eye on him when they knew Bill and I were out. One day Peggy suggested that I remind Craig that if he ever got frightened, hungry or lonely during these times, he was welcome to come over for a visit. By this time, I was a little older and wiser; in other words, I delayed conveying this message to Craig because I knew what his reaction would be. On my birthday Bill and I decided to go out for dinner, leaving Craig alone at home. I alerted Peggy and explained her offer to Craig. And I could just hear the wheels going around in his head. Sure enough, at exactly 8:00 p.m. that evening, after Craig had watched Wheel of Fortune and Jeopardy, he became frightened, hungry, and lonely, and made his visit next door. When we returned to an empty house, I knew exactly where to find Craig. He was ensconced in Jerry's favorite chair, having finished off a soda, chips and ice cream.

As I mentioned earlier, for Craig's 25th birthday we contacted people from the various communities and churches we had known and asked them to acknowledge this special day with a card. He had missed high school graduation, and we hoped to seize this significant event and celebrate. In addition to the 110 cards, he received flowers, balloons, phone calls and gifts. We were overwhelmed. Like young children who play with the boxes and wrapping paper and ignore the gifts, Craig has always been willing to forego gifts and zero in on the greeting cards; he was thrilled. Each and every beloved birthday card was placed in a plastic box and is reviewed daily. In this way he connects with all the people he has known and loved. The box and its

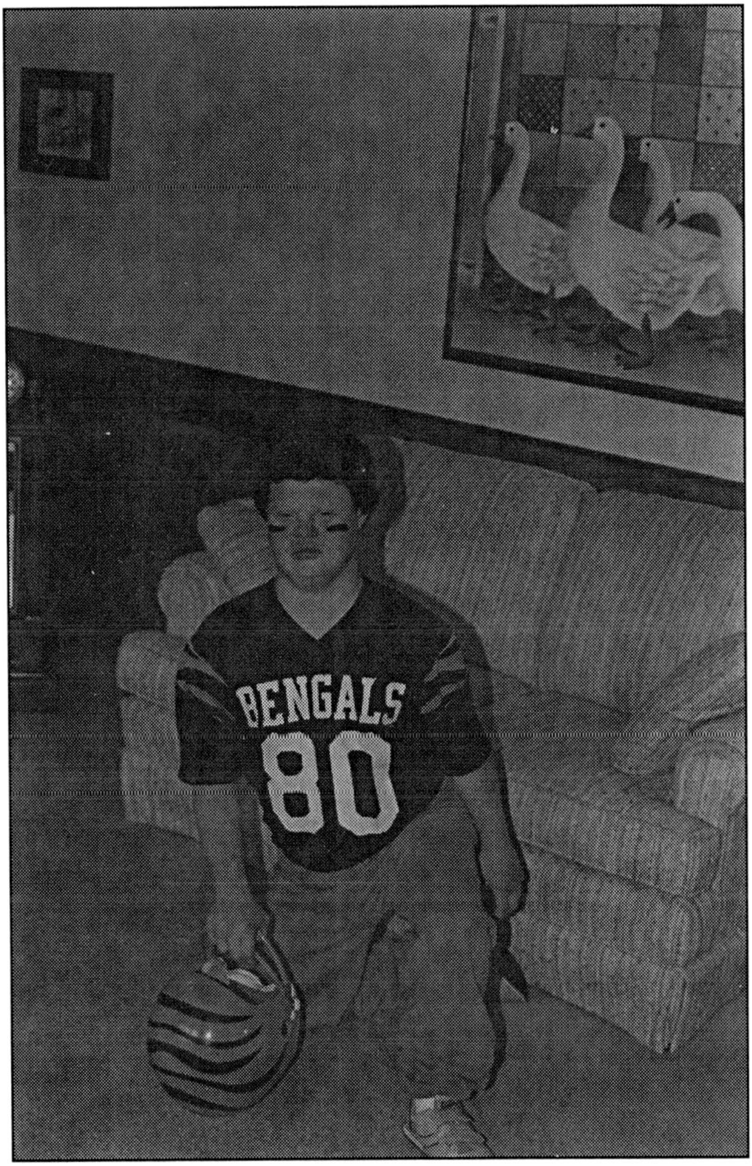

Craig in his favorite team uniform

inventory have grown through the years because he has added every Christmas, Get Well and Birthday card he received. As he sits in his favorite place on the family room floor during his leisure hours, watching endless football games, he is surrounded by reminders of his friendships.

Out of all this has emerged a happy young man with interests in music and sports, especially football, of which he is an avid fan.

Every afternoon after work he slips up to his room, closes the door, and listens to music, singing loudly along with the kids on his tapes and CDs. He possesses a great love for music, pretty good rhythm, and a developing choreography, but as for a musical ear—well, he may have to wait for the heavenly choir for that.

His years with high school peers in Mrs. O's classes, learning to make lunches, have served him well. He packs his lunch for work every day and is content to make his own sandwiches at other times if we are busy. His job, laundry chores, lawn-mowing and woodworking with his dad, raking leaves with his brother, gathering the daily mail and newspaper, his own Sunday school class—all give him a sense of self-worth and independence. Regimen and routine are of great importance to him; in fact, they are his security blankets. He loves to be of help and cooperates fully *if* we lay out our plans ahead of time. He is not spontaneous and cannot be forced into participating in something of which he is unsure. We have learned to carefully time our suggestions and refine our approach.

Thankfully Craig's health has remained strong, though not without some issues. After his hypothyroidism was diagnosed and treatment was begun, Craig grew several inches in stature, which redistributed his weight; yet he remained overweight for a few years. About twenty years ago, I decided to seriously tackle this problem, realizing that I was the one who grocery-shopped, stocked the pantry and dealt out the food. Taking control of his diet, I began making changes—counting calories and fat grams. As the pounds melted off, Craig became increasingly more active and seemingly more alert. The total loss was about thirty pounds, which he has successfully kept off.

Then it was time to tackle allergies. In Virginia Beach and again at Richmond, he was tested to determine his allergies, which were tree and grass pollen, dogs and cats, mold, etc. As of this writing, he is nearing completion of a second round of injections, each round lasting two to three years. Every trip we make to the allergist for injections is very worthwhile. Craig breathes and sleeps better and is, generally, in much better health than before the testing.

Acid reflux is another health issue that seems to plague persons with Down syndrome. After several episodes of choking and difficulty in swallowing, Craig was diagnosed with acid reflux. The treatment with medication, along with dietary restrictions, was established. To date he has had two surgical procedures, which stretched the scar tissue in the esophagus. The swallowing difficulty has nearly ceased; however, we take no chances with tomato-based foods, chocolates, etc. Recently he ate a hamburger for the first time in three years. After a few bites, he softly said, "I just love hamburgers!" He never complains about what he cannot eat, and his attitude makes it easier for us.

Our greatest challenge regarding Craig's illnesses is discovering *where* he hurts. His verbal skills, especially in describing intangibles, are limited. In addition he does not seem to think he should get sick—ever (male hormones?). In fact he gets angry when he does not feel good. Anger, stubbornness and groaning are not good diagnostic tools. Fortunately, we have located great doctors, Dr. Seiler, M.D.and Dr. Breeden, D.D.S., who work respectfully and protectively on his behalf. We feel comfortable calling upon them at any time, and this is a blessing.

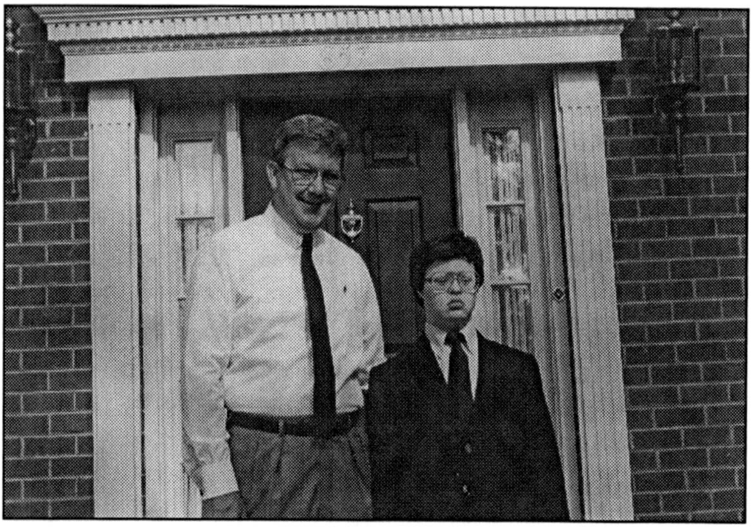

Craig with his father

And so my narrative comes to a close. I hope that you have walked this journey with us, recognizing the struggles and reveling in the successes; I thank you for doing so. Above all, I trust that you have recognized God's love and provision in our life experiences. It is my prayer that they will be an encouragement to you. God bless!

Epilogue

During the course of writing this book, I have referred often to my original goals and purpose: "To illustrate the sustenance and omnipresence of a loving God in the daily living with a special child." I hope I have remained true to that challenge.

The story of Craig's journey is one of sorrow turning into joy. Through God's supplying our daily needs, we emerged from the darkness of 1966 to the light and joy of 2006. Today, I get excited whenever I learn of the birth of a child with Down syndrome because I know there is so much more knowledge, support and acceptance in the world than there was in years past.

I am also thrilled when I hear of parents who use amniocentesis as a diagnostic tool only, and begin preparations to love and nurture the very special child they are about to receive.

> "I praise you because I am fearfully and wonderfully made; your works are wonderful, I know that full well"
>
> —Psalm 139:14 (1)

Endnotes

Prologue

1. Dale Evans Rogers, *Angel Unaware* (New York: Fleming H. Revell Co., 1953).

Chapter 1: The Arrival

1. Proverbs 22:6. (KJV).
2. Mark 10:27. (KJV).

Chapter 2: In My Distress I Cried…

1. "All to Jesus, I Surrender," Words by Judson W. Van DeVenter, music by Winfield S. Weeden. 1896.
2. "Have Thine Own Way, Lord," Words by Adelaide A. Pollard, music by George C. Stebbins. 1907.
3. Elisabeth Kubler-Ross, *On Death and Dying*. Reprinted by Scribner. 1997.
4. Ephesians 5:20. (KJV).
5. Psalms 120:1. (KJV).

Chapter 3: Beginning the Journey

1. "I'll Be a Sunbeam," Words by Nellie Talbot, music by Edwin O. Excell. Circa 1900.

Chapter 4: From the Baby Book

1. Ecclesiastes 3:1. (KJV).
2. Ecclesiastes 3:4. (KJV).

Chapter 6: The Tow-Headed Blue-Eyed Miracle

1. Siegfried M. Pueschel, M.D., Ph.D., J.D., M.P.H., *A Parent's Guide to Down Syndrome,* (Maryland: Paul H. Brookes Publishing Co., 2001). Dr. Pueschel, Professor of Pediatrics at Brown University School of Medicine, and the parent of an adult child with Down syndrome, writes: In 1958, Lejeune discovered that children with Down syndrome had one extra chromosome (in each cell of their bodies), totaling 47 instead of 46. The extra chromosome appears with cell #21–thus the term *trisomy 21.* Subsequently, geneticists detected that individuals with Down syndrome also had other chromosome problems–namely, *translocation* and *mosaicism.* Translocation occurs in only 3% - 4% of children with Down syndrome. In translocation (Craig's diagnosis) the extra chromosome 21 is attached to another chromosome, therefore, there are 46 chromosomes in each cell. It is important to determine whether a child has *translocation* Down syndrome because one of the parents may be a translocation "carrier".

   Therefore, genetic counseling is important because the translocation carrier has an increased risk of having more children with Down syndrome.

Chapter 7: A Bit of Love, a Handshake, a Hug

1. Acts 20:34. (KJV).

Chapter 10: You Know I Hate Meatloaf, and Other Prayers

1. Jerry Boch. *Fiddler on the Roof.* 1964.

Chapter 11: The Balms in Gilead

1. "There Is a Balm in Gilead," Traditional spiritual based on Jeremiah 8:22.

Chapter 12: The Most Important Event of My Life

1. Shriver, Eunice Kennedy. "Athlete Oath." Special Olympics.com. 4 April 2006.

Chapter 13: R-E-T-A-R-D

1. Public Law 94-142, now called Individuals with Disabilities Act (IDEA), passed by congress in 1975. In Order to receive federal funds, states must develop and implement policies that assure a free, appropriate public education to all children with disabilities. The state plans must be consistent with federal statute Title 20. Google.com. 4 April 2006. (2) Matthew 25:40 (KJV).

Epilogue

(1) Psalm 139:14. (NIV).

Readers: Grandma

Printed in the United States
91580LV00002B/14/A

9 781414 108063